WHY CHRISTIANS DIE SICK

AND HOW TO FREE YOURSELF

Amb Promise Ogbonna

E-mail:ontoplifepublishers@gmail.com
E-mail: ambpromiseo@gmail.com

YOU ARE WELCOME TO OUR SPECIAL SERVICES

Weekdays: *12:00-1:00pm. Hour of EmPowerment for All*
Saturdays: *8:00-9:00am. Hour of Healing & Freedom for All*
Sundays: *8:00-9:00am. Hour of Liberty & Restoration for All*
Sundays: *9:00-10:00am. Hour of Kingdom Wealth Transfer for All*
Last Friday Night Monthly: *10:00pm. Night of Restorations for All*
Ambassadors Bible Institute: *Trains and Releases Christ's Ambassadors on His Mission everywhere! Enroll today!*

Venue: 24 Independence Street, Behind O'MARK Schools by O'MARK Bus Stop, LASU Road, Igando Lagos.

Contents

First Words

Chapters

<u>*OUR HEAVENLY MANDATE*</u>

To Preach The Everlasting Gospel to All everywhere, Stop anything after man's destruction, Bring Healing, Liberty and Restoration to all; Raise, Build and Plant All as Christ's Ambassadors on His Living Mission everywhere and Restore all things!

WHY BELIEVERS DIE SICK
AND HOW TO FREE YOURSELF

Christians are God's children redeemed with the Precious Blood of Jesus Christ. They should be like Christ in every way but are dying sick just like any body else in spite of God's love for them. It is not supposed to be so. Nevertheless, it is happening and happening at an alarming rate.

Why is it so? Why is the most treasured possession of God the Father suffering and ending like the heathen – in shame and reproaches? What has brought so low God's greatly esteemed and highly prized inheritance?

This Publication which is God's mind revealed shows why and also how to free yourself, your loved ones and everyone else around you.

It is packaged to enable you maximize God's ability in you to be able to fulfill you life's purpose and arrive destination in colour and dignity. God bless you as you discover and help others see the light.

CHAPTER 1

BEWARE OF WHAT YOU HEAR!

You are word made! Whatever you are presently, words made you to be.

You are made up of words. That's why you are a spirit.

John 6:63 "It is the Spirit who gives life; the flesh profits nothing. The words that I speak to you are spirit, and they are life."
John 3:6 "That which is born of the flesh is flesh, and that which is born of the Spirit is spirit."
John 1:12-13

12 But as many as received Him, to them He gave the right to become children of God, to those who believe in His name:

13 who were born, not of blood, nor of the will of the flesh, nor of the will of man, but of God.

John 10:35 "He called them gods, to whom the word of God came (and the Scripture cannot be broken).

John 1:1-3

1 ¶ In the beginning was the Word, and the Word was with God, and the Word was God.

2 He was in the beginning with God.

3 All things were made through Him, and without Him nothing was made that was made.

God is The Word. God is Spirit!

Wrong words Causes Sickness and Destroys

Words make you or break you. You are made up of words. Beware of what you hear! Who you listen to and what you hear determines what happens in your life and to you. Don't die sick by feeding yourself with poisonous words that ruin and destroy you. You are Word composite. So mind what you feed yourself.

Ignorance Causes Sickness and Destroys

Psalm 82:5-7

5 They know not neither will they understand; they walk on in darkness. All the foundations of the earth are gone out of course.

6 I have said, ye are gods; and all of you are children of the most High.

7 But ye shall die like men and fall like one of the princes.

Ignorance, lack of knowledge and understanding will lead ultimately to captivity, bondage, prison, walking in darkness and a tearing or falling apart of everything that God or man had put in place on earth; and will lead to sickness, death and destruction of the individuals. "GODS or children of the Most High can die like men and fall like one of the princes.

Poverty Causes Sickness and Destroys

Proverbs 10:15 "The destruction of the poor is their poverty."

Psalm 34:6 "This poor man called, and the Lord heard him; he saved him out of all his troubles." (NIV)

Psalm 118:25 "Save now, I beseech thee, o Lord: O Lord, I beseech thee, SEND NOW PROSPERITY." (KJV)

But the poor man cried or called to the Lord and He heard him and SAVED him from all his Troubles. Until and unless the Lord saves the poor from HIS POVERTY, he is not saved.

The destruction of the poor cannot end until he is saved from his poverty. That means, prosperity is a must to maintain healing and health. And prosperity from the Lord is what puts to an end the wasting and destruction of the poor.

How do you attain to God's Kind of Prosperity and Enforce Your Healing and Health?

- Hear God's Word. Listen to the Word of God always even when you don't feel like it. Proverbs 4:20-22
- Think and Meditate on God's Word. Joshua 1:8; Psalm 1:2-3
- Keep God's Word in your heart. Psalm 119:9-11; Proverbs 4:21-23
- Speak God's Word always. Joshua 1:8; Proverbs 18:20-21
- Give God all His Tithe. Malachi 3:7-11
- Sow your seed even when in need. Psalm 126:4-6; Proverbs 3:9-10
- Love and Praise God always. Mark 12:30; Hebrews 13:15-16
- Get involved in the Gospel Business at all cost and by all means. Luke 12:32-33; Matthew 6:33
- Always be thankful to the LORD. Psalm 92:1-2; 1 Thessalonians 5:18

This knowledge and understanding is so important because it is the only surety for the salvation of the poor from their sickness, poverty, poverty, and destructions.

CHAPTER 2

GOD DOESN'T WANT YOU SICK

The Lord God healed All in the past to show you what He is still committed to in the present.

Psalm 107:20 "He sent His Word and *Healed them* and delivered them from their destructions."

Acts 10:38 "How **God** anointed Jesus of Nazareth with the Holy Spirit and with power, who **went about** doing good and **healing all** who were oppressed by the devil, for God was with Him."

The Lord God is the same Healer Always

Exodus 3:14 "And God said to Moses, "I AM WHO I AM." And He said, "Thus you shall say to the children of Israel, 'I AM has sent me to you.'"

Hebrew 13:8 "Jesus Christ is the same yesterday, today, and forever."

The LORD (the Healer) doesn't change

Malachi 3:6 "For I am the LORD, I do not change..."

John 14:7,9-11

7 "If you had known Me, you would have known My Father also; and from now on you know Him and have seen Him."
9 …He who has seen Me has seen the Father
10 "Do you not believe that I am in the Father, and the Father in Me? The words that I speak to you I do not speak on My own authority; but the Father who dwells in Me does the works.
11 "Believe Me that I am in the Father and the Father in Me, or else believe Me for the sake of the works themselves.

The LORD is out to destroy sickness.

Psalm 107:20 "He sent His Word and Healed them and delivered them from their destructions."

1John 3:8
8 He who sins is of the devil, for the devil has sinned from the beginning. For this purpose the Son of God was manifested, that He might destroy the works of the devil.

Exodus 15:26 and said, "If you diligently heed the voice of the LORD your God and do what is right in His sight, give ear to His commandments and keep all His statutes, I will put none of the diseases on you which I have brought on the Egyptians. For I am the LORD who heals you."

God doesn't want You sick.
3John 2 Beloved, I pray that you may prosper in all things and be in health, just as your soul prospers.

God doesn't want The Sick to perish.

2 Peter 3:9 ¶ The Lord is not slack concerning His promise, as some count slackness, but is longsuffering toward us, not willing that any should perish but that all should come to repentance.
Psalm 107:20 "He sent His Word and Healed them and delivered them from their destructions."

God Sends and Approves of His Servants through Healing Miracles to free the Sick
Acts 2:22 "Men of Israel, hear these words: Jesus of Nazareth, a Man attested by God to you by miracles, wonders, and signs which God did through Him in your midst, as you yourselves also know--

Acts 5:12,15,16
12 ¶ And through the hands of the apostles many signs and wonders were done among the people.
15 so that they brought the sick out into the streets and laid them on beds and couches, that at least the shadow of Peter passing by might fall on some of them.
 16 Also a multitude gathered from the surrounding cities to Jerusalem, bringing sick people and those who were tormented by unclean spirits, and they were all healed.

2 Corinthians 12:12 "Truly the signs of an apostle were accomplished among you with all perseverance, in signs and wonders and mighty deeds."

Hebrews 2:4 "God also bearing witness both with signs and wonders, with various miracles, and gifts of the Holy Spirit, according to His own will."

Psalm 107:20 "He sent His Word and Healed them and delivered them from their destructions."

Proverbs 13:17
17 ¶ A wicked messenger falls into trouble, But a faithful ambassador brings health.

We are here to publish, spread or distribute His healing and health to everyone.

CHAPTER 3
WHY BELIEVERS DIE SICK

On the 15th of March 2006, the Lord again showed me why believers die cheaply at the hands of the enemy because of sickness and disease.

No believer who follows God obediently CAN or WILL BE ALLOWED TO DIE by God through sickness. God is committed fully to performing His Word.

In Jeremiah 1:12 The LORD says "I will watch over my words to perform it."

Why Born Again Believers are Dying Sick

God sustains all things by The Living Word. *Hebrew 1:3, "Who being the brightness of His glory and the express image of His person, and upholding all things by the word of His power."* That means, our hedge of protection is kept secured by The Living Word. God created us by His Word. God made us by the Word. God keeps or preserves us by the Word. God is upholding everything by the Word of His Power. Therefore, whoever breaks the hedge or whoever fails to keep, do or live by the Word, a serpent will bite him.

Ecclesiastes 10:8 "He who digs a pit will fall into it, And whoever breaks through a wall will be bitten by a serpent."

Believers are dying sick because they are breaking the Word of the Covenant!

Numbers 21:4-9
4 ¶ Then they journeyed from Mount Hor by the Way of the Red Sea, to go around the land of Edom; and the soul of the people became very discouraged on the way.
 5 And the people spoke against God and against Moses: "Why have you brought us up out of Egypt to die in the wilderness? For there is no food and no water, and our soul loathes this worthless bread."
 6 So the LORD sent fiery serpents among the people, and they bit the people; and many of the people of Israel died.
 7 Therefore the people came to Moses, and said, "We have sinned, for we have spoken against the LORD and against you; pray to the LORD that He take away the serpents from us." So Moses prayed for the people.

8 Then the LORD said to Moses, "Make a fiery serpent, and set it on a pole; and it shall be that everyone who is bitten, when he looks at it, shall live."
9 So Moses made a bronze serpent, and put it on a pole; and so it was, if a serpent had bitten anyone, when he looked at the bronze serpent, he lived.

It is the breaking of the covenant by believers that is solely responsible for the death of believers through sickness.

God cannot break His Covenant or Word

Psalm 89:34 "My covenant I will not break, Nor alter the word that has gone out of My lips."

John 10:35 "…the Word of God… the Scripture cannot be broken."
What is the command of the Lord that
Believers must obey to be healed? What is
God's Key to Being Sick Free and Healthy By the Believer?

James 5:14-15,19-20
14 Is anyone among you sick/ Let him call for the elders of the Church, and let them pray over him, anointing him with oil in the name of the Lord.
15 And the prayer of faith will save the sick, and the Lord will (unfailingly) raise him up. And if he has committed sins, he will be forgiven.
19 Brethren, if anyone among you wanders from the truth, and someone turns him back,

20 let him know that he who turns a sinner from the error of his way will save a soul from death and cover a multitude of sins.

The church is not to record a single death among her members as s result of sickness, illness or disease or bodily affliction. Christian Believers are not permitted by God to die by any kind of sickness. That means, no deadly disease or sickness, no matter how deadly it is or may appear to be has the power to take or claim the life of the believer if we know what God expects us to do and we willingly obey Him and do them.

That means, HIV/AIDS, Cancer or Tuberculosis etc has no power to cause the death of the believer, even the believer who fell into sin. This is solely talking about believers who are born again. No matter the cause of the sickness or disease, God has made a provision for your healing. And when you obey and do as He commands, there is no force on earth that is working against you to destroy you through sickness that will have the power to kill you. The death of the believer is never to be decided by the devil or sickness. This is why I am most certain that no member of the church I pastor will die premature or untimely because of sickness if they only hear, believe and do as I am sent to tell and teach them. Listen to me: there is no sickness or disease that has the power to cut short your life by any means if you hear, believe and fully obey the word of the Lord He sent me to show you.

What is God's Provision for the Healing of the Believer?

Let's look at James 5:14-15 again. God says:
James 5:14-15

14 "Is anyone AMONG YOU sick? Let him call for the Elders (Pastors or Shepherds) of the church, and let them pray over him, anointing him with oil in the name of the Lord.
15 And the prayer of faith will save the sick, and the Lord will raise him up. And if he has committed sins, he will be forgiven."

James' epistle is for professing believers only as *"Among you"* clearly shows. "Let him call the Elders of the church" shows that he must belong to (a particular) 'church' or 'assembly' of God's people. James 5:14-15 is not for unbelievers but for believers only, those believers who are sick. "Is any among you sick, let him call for the Elders of the church."
The Word shows that God expects every sick believer (Born again Christian) to SEEK HIM FIRST for Healing if ever sick. No matter the sickness, no matter the cause of the sickness, God demands we live and walk with Him by faith and secure His healing by His ordained spiritual means. God never wants us to seek man first until we have sought Him.

Exodus 15:26, "I am the LORD who heals you."

God says, *"I am the Lord your Healer."*
In James 5:14-15, He says, *"Is anyone among you sick, Let him call for the Elders of the church."*
Note: *God never said you go get, look for or call for any other man or person in the church other than the Elders.* He specifically said who to call. To do something else or call someone else is simply disobedience and is a costly mistake to make.

The Lord knows there could be medical experts in the church yet He wants His children to hear and obey His Word if they ever have any health challenges. This necessarily does not mean that there is no basis to use or seek the advice of medical practitioners. But it is absolutely contrary to God's Word for any believer, who is sick to call for or seek for any human medical help, without first seeking for divine help from God Himself through His appointed and ordained elders, pastors, or ministers in the church. Those who ignore the LORD and His ways end up suffering or dying. This is why it is important for you to be in a church where your Leaders preach the full gospel that builds faith and enables obedience.

Please take responsibility and go to where you will be told the whole truth or where you will hear the full gospel if not you will suffer terribly and might end killed and destroyed by the enemy with sickness or disease. And at the end of your life you will still be judged for doing wrong and ending wrongly.

What is the full Gospel?

God's greatest wish is for you to have complete prosperity or total wellbeing.

3 John 2, "Beloved, I pray that you may prosper in all things and be in health, just as your soul prospers."

Therefore the full gospel is that which addresses every area of man's need with valid proofs.

Romans 15:18-20

18 For I will not dare to speak of any of those things which Christ has not accomplished through me, in word and deed, to make the Gentiles obedient--

19 in mighty signs and wonders, by the power of the Spirit of God, so that from Jerusalem and round about to Illyricum I have fully preached the gospel of Christ.

20 And so I have made it my aim to preach the gospel

1 Corinthians 4:20 "For the kingdom of God is not in word but in power."

1 Corinthians 2:4-5

4 And my speech and my preaching were not with persuasive words of human wisdom, but in demonstration of the Spirit and of power,

5 that your faith should not be in the wisdom of men but in the power of God.

Matthew 4:23-24

23 ¶ And Jesus went about all Galilee, teaching in their synagogues, preaching the gospel of the kingdom, and healing all kinds of sickness and all kinds of disease among the people.

24 Then His fame went throughout all Syria; and they brought to Him all sick people who were afflicted with various diseases and torments, and those who were demon-possessed, epileptics, and paralytics; and He healed them.

Luke 6:17-19

17 And He came down with them and stood on a level place with a crowd of His disciples and a great multitude of people from all Judea and Jerusalem, and from the

seacoast of Tyre and Sidon, who came to hear Him and be healed of their diseases,

18 as well as those who were tormented with unclean spirits. And they were healed.

19 And the whole multitude sought to touch Him, for power went out from Him and healed them all.

Luke 7:13-15,18-20

13 When the Lord saw her, He had compassion on her and said to her, "Do not weep."

14 Then He came and touched the open coffin, and those who carried him stood still. And He said, "Young man, I say to you, arise."

15 So he who was dead sat up and began to speak. And He presented him to his mother.

18 Then the disciples of John reported to him concerning all these things.

19 ¶ And John, calling two of his disciples to him, sent them to Jesus, saying, "Are You the Coming One, or do we look for another?"

20 When the men had come to Him, they said, "John the Baptist has sent us to You, saying, 'Are You the Coming One, or do we look for another?'"

21 And that very hour He cured many of infirmities, afflictions, and evil spirits; and to many blind He gave sight.

22 Jesus answered and said to them, "Go and tell John the things you have seen and heard: that the blind see, the lame walk, the lepers are cleansed, the deaf hear, the dead are raised, the poor have the gospel preached to them.

They suffer terribly that ignore God

Mark 5:25-26

25 Now a certain woman had a flow of blood for twelve years,

26 and had suffered many things from many physicians. She had spent all that she had and was no better, but rather grew worse.

Jeremiah 14:19 "Have You utterly rejected Judah? Has Your soul loathed Zion? Why have You stricken us so that there is no healing for us? We looked for peace, but there was no good; And for the time of healing, and there was trouble.

Men suffered and Died that ignore God

1. *2 Kings 1:2-4,6,16-17*

2 Now Ahaziah fell through the lattice of his upper room in Samaria, and was injured; so he sent messengers and said to them, "Go, inquire of Baal-Zebub, the god of Ekron, whether I shall recover from this injury."

3 But the angel of the LORD said to Elijah the Tishbite, "Arise, go up to meet the messengers of the king of Samaria, and say to them, 'Is it because there is no God in Israel that you are going to inquire of Baal-Zebub, the god of Ekron?'

4 "Now therefore, thus says the LORD: 'You shall not come down from the bed to which you have gone up, but you shall surely die.'"

6 So they said to him, "A man came up to meet us, and said to us, 'Go, return to the king who sent you, and say to him, "Thus says the LORD: 'Is it because there is no God in Israel that you are sending to inquire of Baal-Zebub, the god of Ekron? Therefore you shall not come down from

the bed to which you have gone up, but you shall surely die."'"

16 Then he said to him, "Thus says the LORD: 'Because you have sent messengers to inquire of Baal-Zebub, the god of Ekron, is it because there is no God in Israel to inquire of His word? Therefore you shall not come down from the bed to which you have gone up, but you shall surely die.'"

17 So Ahaziah died according to the word of the LORD which Elijah had spoken.

2. *2Chronicles 16:12-13*

12 And in the thirty-ninth year of his reign, Asa became diseased in his feet, and his malady was severe; yet in his disease he did not seek the LORD, but the physicians.

13 So Asa rested with his fathers; he died in the forty-first year of his reign.

3. *Jeremiah 46:11*

"In vain you will use many medicines; You shall not be cured."

4. *Jeremiah 30:13*

"There is no one to plead your cause, That you may be bound up; You have no healing medicines."

God Cannot Fail To Heal All That Trust in Him

"Thou wilt keep him in perfect peace, whose mind is stayed on thee: because he trusteth in thee." *Isaiah 26:3*

"Trust in the Lord with all thine heart; and lean not unto thy own understanding." *Proverbs 3:5*

"And call upon me in the day of trouble: I will deliver thee, and thou shall glorify me." *Psalm 50:15*

Today, most believers who fall sick immediately go for their doctors or the best hospitals ignoring God's command to call for the elders of the church. Every believer who does so is guilty of direct disobedience against the command, statute, word or ordinance of God as clearly stated in the scripture.

James 5:14-15

14 Is anyone among you sick? Let him call for the elders of the church, and let them pray over him, anointing him with oil in the name of the Lord.

15 And the prayer of faith will save the sick, and the Lord will raise him up. And if he has committed sins, he will be forgiven.

The body of Christ fails to realize that God who knows the end from the beginning made His provisions for His people bearing in mind that doctors and health specialists will one day emerge. God's Word is settled forever in heaven and cannot be changed no matter what happens on earth. The ignorance of God's provisions and disobedience to His command has plunged many believers into bondage to the ways of the world. This is why most sick believers are being destroyed by the enemy through sickness that God wants to heal to glorify His name when His people obey His word.

The Living Word says: Is anyone among you sick? Let him call for the elders of the church..." That means any believer who falls sick of any sickness or disease and who, instead of calling for the elders of the church, calls for the doctor is guilty of total disobedience and so opens himself/herself up for the enemy to kill and destroy through disobedience. The doctors are not at fault and should not be blamed for this abnormality. No doctor has ever bothered me since 31st May 1991 when the LORD took me and showed me this secret. The body of Christ because of her ignorance has caused God much pain as it were. But the time has come for us to rise and take delivery of what is ours. The LORD our Healer is Our Maker and knows us completely and is the best Consultant and Physician to handle any of our health challenges. You must begin to consult Him.

When sick believers defiantly or ignorantly call their doctors, they plainly tell God, they don't need Him and don't believe in Him or His Word.

They show God that He is not capable of healing their diseases or handle their cases. They tell God He is not a true loving God who can keep His Word by doing what He says. They tell God they don't trust in Him to make good His Word but trust in man to heal them. They show God they don't need His guidance, counsel, advice or wisdom but rather prefer the guidance, counsel, advice or wisdom of men. They show God to His face, that He is a liar as they don't believe He can do what He says by healing them. So they abandon God who created them and go to man who cannot do anything. So many of them never return from their sick beds. Some return having the number of their years or days cut short. If the enemy is allowed to steal anything from you, he has been allowed to remove something from your life. Therefore, to cut him off, God shows us the way. He says: "call the Elders of the church, and let them pray over him (the sick) anointing him with oil in the name of the Lord. And the prayer of faith will save the sick, and the Lord will raise him up. And if he has committed sins, he will be forgiven." And God cannot lie (Titus 1:2); Let God be true and all men liars (Romans 3:4). He will not alter his Word (Psalm 89:34), but must perform the Word that has gone forth out of His mouth in righteousness (Isaiah 45:23; 55:10-11, Jeremiah 1:12). For "Forever His Word is settled in heaven" (Psalm 119:89).

James 5:14-15 shows the basic fundamental truth about the believers healing from all sicknesses.

- Sickness is not to be common among believers.
- There is healing for any believer who is sick no matter the sickness, regardless of the cause of it.
- There is the God-ordained way for the believer's healing.
- The sick is to call FIRST (and only) for the church's Elders.
- The church's Elders must believe in Christ the healer.
- The church's Elders must believe in divine healing.
- The church's Elders must believe in the prayer of faith.
- The church's Elders must believe in the Anointing with oil and always carry it and be willing to administer it when called upon.
- The sick must also be taught on divine healing and Christ as the healer and on the Anointing oil.
- The sick must believe in the Anointing with oil.
- The sick must be taught on Faith in Christ as the Healer.

- The sick must believe in divine Healing and go for it.
- The sick believer must know the result of obedience - Healing no matter the sickness or its cause - and seeking God.
- The sick believer must also know the consequences of disobedience and seeking medical help first and not God or before him - suffering, death/destruction.
- Believers must be taught the truth and reliability on God who cannot fail rather than man.
- Believers must be taught to confidently obey The Living Word and expect God to do all He says He will do.

This is very important. If by being willing and obedient we eat the good of the land according to Isaiah 1:19, it also follows that by being unwilling and disobedient we face the wrath of the Lord and partake of the evil upon the land (earth) which includes among others sickness, poverty, evils, curses, etc.

**Disobedience, caused mostly by unbelief,
Is sin and its wages is death**

1Samuel 15:22-23
22 Then Samuel said: "Has the LORD as great delight in burnt offerings and sacrifices, As in obeying the voice of the LORD? Behold, to obey is better than sacrifice, And to heed than the fat of rams.
 23 For rebellion is as the sin of witchcraft, And stubbornness is as iniquity and idolatry. Because you have rejected the word of the LORD, He also has rejected you from being king."
Romans 14:23, "for whatever is not from faith is sin."

Romans 6:23 "For the wages of sin is death, but the gift of God is eternal life in Christ Jesus our Lord."

Most believers that have health challenges today run to human beings (medical practitioners) because they believe in them or have faith in them rather than run to God through His Word and ordained channels (the Elders) for their healings. This is because they have been made to see and believe in man who they see more than they believe in The LORD.

Ecclesiastes 3:14 shows it is only what the Lord does that lasts forever, nothing can be added to it or anything taken from it because God does it so that men should fear before Him. Any "healing" effected by man is temporary, unreal, and only time will prove it so; and a most certain way to premature death. So why waste your resources and life on that which cannot will not last?

Even if man succeeds in effecting a relief, the reason for sickness which is sin or a breach of the covenant regulations has not been dealt with. Until the tree is uprooted, cutting off of the leaves or its fruits is doing absolutely nothing if one desires to terminate the tree. It is just a matter of time, the same leaves and fruits will grow up again for as long as the tree is not uprooted. So all forms of human, medical provisions for man's healing is a waste of time, resources and life in comparison to that which the LORD has made and ordained for us His chosen ones. Just like a tree branch naturally grows from its place, sickness or death will still naturally result from the same sickness that man has tried to cut down. This is because sickness is spiritual and of the devil and cannot be handled by man's mere methods. Any sickness cut down by man will grow again because the disease-germ causing it, which temporarily went into hiding when it encountered an enemy, will come up sooner or later.

But when the sick believer accepts The Living Word of God and calls for the Elders of the church and they pray over him, anointing him with oil in the name of the Lord (Jesus Christ), the prayer of faith will save, heal, deliver, emancipate, recover, make whole, preserve in total soundness the sick, and the Lord will raise him up. And if he has committed sins, he will be forgiven.

That means, God will ultimately and completely deal with the root-cause of the sickness so that there will be no future occurrence. Once the tree is uprooted, cast away and destroyed, it can never sprout, grow, bear leaves and produce fruits again. So to achieve the perpetual healing of sickness in the believer's life, it is absolutely important to follow the ordained way of the Lord who is the creator and maker of the believer. If this is not done every effort of man to cut off and destroy sickness is nothing worthwhile.

James 5:14-15 is God's complete and absolute remedy for the believer who falls sick. That means whatever illness, plague, sickness or disease that befalls the believer will and must give way as the believer obeys The Living Word of God by calling Elders of the church who know and believe in God's provision for the saints and are willing and ready to obey it absolutely.

Faith-prayer and anointing with oil is the way out for the believer.

Believers cannot set aside God's statutes, commands, ordinances, testimonies or Word for their healing and not face the consequences of their acts of disobedience.

Your Obedience to His Word Shows Your Love for Him and Commits Him

Psalm 91:14-16 (KJV)
14 Because he hath set his love upon me, therefore will I deliver him: I will set him on high, because he hath known my name.
15 He shall call upon me, and I will answer him: I will be with him in trouble; I will deliver him, and honour him.
16 With long life will I satisfy him, and show him my salvation.

Premature, untimely death through sickness, illness, or disease is never God's plan. God wants to heal your body so that He can preserve you blameless spirit, and soul, and body; whether you are in the city or in the field, in your going out and in your coming in from this time forth and forevermore in Jesus Name.

1Thessalonians 5:23-24
23 ¶ Now may the God of peace Himself sanctify you completely; and may your whole spirit, soul, and body be preserved blameless at the coming of our Lord Jesus Christ.
24 He who calls you is faithful, who also will do it.

Deuteronomy 28:3,6
3 "Blessed shall you be in the city, and blessed shall you be in the country.

6 "Blessed shall you be when you come in, and blessed shall you be when you go out.

Psalm 121:7-8
7 The LORD shall preserve you from all evil; He shall preserve your soul.
 8 The LORD shall preserve your going out and your coming in From this time forth, and even forevermore.

Believers must be a part and parcel of His body (the church) and the Pastors, Ministers and Elders in our midst must ever know, believe and be ready, willing and obedient to the teaching of Scripture to minister healing to anyone who is sick and calls for them.
Please note: Believers must be taught to call for the Pastors, Ministers, Elders, and Leaders of the church first as they used to call for their doctors anytime they are sick. The Ministers must also know that once there is a call from anyone who is sick among us, they are to go and anoint the sick with oil in the Name of the LORD and pray the prayer of faith over the sick. Once they do so, the prayer of faith made coupled with anointing the sick with oil in the Name of the Lord Jesus Christ will save the sick from whatever sickness he may be suffering, and the Lord will raise him up [from his sick bed or point of death or even of death]. And if he has committed sins, he will be forgiven.

Anointing the Sick with Oil Precedes the Prayer of Faith

"Is anyone among you sick? Let him call for the elders of the church, and let them pray over him anointing him with oil in the Name of the Lord..." shows very clearly that

God wants believers to belong to a congregation of His Saints and be committed in such a way that the Leaders, Elders, or Pastors of the assembly of God's people will know him or be known by them.

Involvement and service in His House qualifies you for God's Healing

Believers are to get involved in the congregation where they belong and serve God well. Commitment to service is what makes the Ministers or Elders know him/her.

The anointing with oil which The Lord commands is to be done by faith in the knowledge that the Holy Spirit shall impart God's life and healing to the body of the sick and raise him up.

Romans 8:11 The Spirit that raised Jesus from the dead will, via the anointing with oil in the Name of the Lord will work in the sick and gives them life in their bodies, and so raise them from sickness and death.

Anointing the Sick with Oil is an Act of Faith

The anointing oil is used symbolically by faith. It is the obedience, act of faith and declaration by the elders that commits the Lord to act and save the sick. The Holy Spirit gives life to the bodies of the sick and declares them free from sickness as the Word is spoken. That means when the elders speak the word of faith and anoint the sick with oil in the name of the Lord (James 5:14-15; Romans 8:11), life is imparted into the sick by The Holy Spirit and the sick is saved and raised up just as Jesus was raised up by The Holy Spirit (Romans 8:11).

Romans 10:6-8
6 But the righteousness of faith speaks in this way, "Do not say in your heart, 'Who will ascend into heaven?'" (that is, to bring Christ down from above)
 7 or," 'Who will descend into the abyss?'" (that is, to bring Christ up from the dead).
 8 But what does it say? "The word is near you, in your mouth and in your heart" (that is, the word of faith which we preach):

2 Timothy 1:10, "Our Savior Jesus Christ, who has abolished death and brought life and immortality to light through the gospel."

2 Corinthians 4:10-11
10 always carrying about in the body the dying of the Lord Jesus, that the life of Jesus also may be manifested in our body.
 11 For we who live are always delivered to death for Jesus' sake, that the life of Jesus also may be manifested in our mortal flesh.

Therefore it is clear that the Anointing with oil is a way of imparting the divine, God-kind of life, health and strength to the sick by The Holy Spirit.

Anointing the Sick with Oil is a New Testament Ordinance

The ordinance of anointing the sick with oil is God's appointed and ordained act of faith through which God's Spirit, life, health, strength and power is infused into the mortal body of the sick by The Holy Spirit. And this is the God's ordained way for the sick believer to be healed totally and completely with the root cause of the sickness cu off.

The Elders of the church are to pray the prayer of faith and anoint the sick believer, on the invitation of the sick, with the anointing oil in the Name of the Lord and the prayer of faith will save the sick and the Lord will raise him up and if he has committed sins, he will be forgiven. Any sick believer who is sick or dies as a result of sickness suffers or dies primarily for rejecting this ordinance, statute, or command of God.

Believers are not to call medical doctors but the Elders of the church as God ordained and they are to respond immediately by going with the Anointing oil to the sick. On arrival, they are to pray the prayer of faith and anoint the sick with oil in the name of the Lord. And the prayer of faith will save the sick and the Lord will raise him up (the sick believer by the LORD Himself). And if he has committed sins, he will be forgiven.

Sick Believers Are Anointed With Oil While Sick Unbelievers Are Laid Hands On

The sick believer is not to be laid hands on as the Lord Commands to be done for the unbelievers in Mark 16:15-18.

The laying on of hands is not for the sick believer but the sick unbeliever (mankind without Christ or those who are not born again).

Mark 16:15-18 believers are sent into the entire world TO PREACH THE GOSPEL OF THE KINGDOM AND TO LAY HANDS ON THE SICK. "And these signs shall follow them…" they are to lay hands on the sick (newly converted and unbelievers) and they shall recover. The laying on of hands on the sick is to be used to authenticate the preaching of the gospel in areas and places in the world where the gospel has not reached or been preached.

The disciples did so

Mark 16:20, "They went and preached everywhere, the Lord working with them and confirming the word through the accompanying signs. Amen.

Paul did so

Acts 28:8-9 (NIV)

8 It happened that the father of Publius lay sick with fever and dysentery, and Paul visited him and prayed, and putting his hands on him healed him.

9 And when this has taken place, the rest of the people in the island who had diseases also came and were cured.

Paul got to the Island of Malta (Melita) and by laying on of hands healed the sick who were there. Paul fully preached the gospel with power and signs followed.

Romans 15:18-19

18 For I will not dare to speak of any of those things which Christ has not accomplished through me, in word and deed, to make the Gentiles obedient--

19 in mighty signs and wonders, by the power of the Spirit of God, so that from Jerusalem and round about to Illyricum I have fully preached the gospel of Christ.

2 Corinthians 12:12, "Truly the signs of an apostle were accomplished among you with all perseverance, in signs and wonders and mighty deeds."

Hebrews 2:4, "God also bearing witness both with signs and wonders, with various miracles, and gifts of the Holy Spirit, according to His own will?"

Laying on of hands in the Name of Jesus is primarily for unbelievers, the unconverted ones or for those who have newly come to the Christian faith or have been established in the faith as a believer or as member of a church assembly.

Note the Lord's word:

They will lay hands on the sick, and THEY WILL RECOVER

No one I lay hands on in His Name will fail to recover no matter the Sickness. The Lord said so, I believe it and that settles it. That means "the sick will get well" or "they will be well" when the believers lay hands on the unconverted or the newly born again people in every place in the world -"everywhere".

Note: When hands are laid on the sick, The Lord Himself goes into work in diverse ways - as he chooses to bring healing and recovery to the sick.

1Corinthians 12:6 says "There are diversities of activities or operations, but   it is the same God who works all in all."

That means, when believers lay hands on the sick, the Lord Himself works on each individual case to effect a healing. He might not do it the same way always. He has diversities of activities or operations to get man healed but all is subject to our obedience to His instructions. It is not the duty of the believer to effect a cure but to lay hands on the sick. It is not the duty of the Lord to lay hands on the sick but to effect a cure/heal. Man (the believer) has his duty. The Lord has His own duty and responsibility. It is the believer's duty to obey the command to lay hands on the sick. It is the duty of The Lord who works all in all to effect a cure or heal the sick.

By laying hands on the sick, the believer who carries the supernatural healing virtue, power, ability or life of God passes on to the sick what he carries and God Himself takes over and by His Spirit, Life and Power operates or acts and healing results.

The laying on of hands is an act of faith in the one who commands us to lay hands on the sick and they shall recover, be made well or healed. So we obey the Lord and lay hands on the sick and the Lord takes over and confirms His Word with the sign of healing following.

Mark 16:18-20
18 "they will take up serpents; and if they drink anything deadly, it will by no means hurt them; they will lay hands on the sick, and they will recover."

19 ¶ So then, after the Lord had spoken to them, He was received up into heaven, and sat down at the right hand of God.

20 And they went out and preached everywhere, the Lord working with them and confirming the word through the accompanying signs. Amen.

"They shall lay hands on the sick and they shall recover" shows that most certainly, recovery is inevitable but how long it will be before it is manifested is not stated. That means, even if there is no dramatic, immediate change or result after hands have been laid, the believer must believe in the God of The Living Word and know that Scriptures cannot be broken.(John10:35). Therefore, once hands have been laid on the sick, they should begin to thank and praise the Lord for He cannot fail to do as He said.

CHAPTER 4

FAITH IN GOD'S WORD PRECEDES HEALING

Faith in the Word is a necessity for healing to happen.

"My covenant I will not break, Nor alter the word that has gone out of My lips."

Psalm 89:34

"Then the LORD said to me, "You have seen well, for I am ready to perform My word."
Jeremiah 1:12

That means, whether there is instant miraculous and dramatic physical manifestation of healing or not, there must not be any doubt as to the truth, reality and infallibility of God's Word. God will do all He promised. The sick will recover after we have laid hands on them, no matter the sickness or the cause of it. This shows that HIV/AIDS, cancer, tumor, blindness, deafness, all manner of sickness and all manner of disease must be healed by the faithful obedience of believers to the commandment of the Lord. God's faithfulness is committed when we obey His word and lay hands on the sick.

1 Thessalonians 5:24 "He who calls you is faithful, who also will do it."

Therefore, whether the healing is spontaneous or gradual, we must never doubt or waiver at The Lord's ability to do as He has said.

In Numbers 21:4-9 - All who believed and obeyed the Word were healed.

John3:14-16 shows that all who believe and obey The Living Word will be saved and healed.

Isaiah 45:22 - Turn to Me and be saved all the ends of the earth for I am God, And there is no other.

Exodus 15:26 - I am the Lord that healeth thee.

Acts 10:38 - How God anointed Jesus of Nazareth (not of Heaven) with the   Holy Ghost and with power who went about doing good and healing all who were oppressed of the devil; for God was with Him.

Malachi 3:6 - I am the Lord I change not so you cannot be consumed by that Sickness.

Hebrew 13:8 - Jesus Christ the same (Healer) always, even for evermore.

Psalm 107:20 - He sent His word and healed them and delivered them from   their destructions.

Psalm 68:11 - The Lord gave the word, great is the company of those who publish it.

Proverbs 4:20-22 - The Living Word is life and health to all their flesh.

Hebrew 4:12-13 - The Living Word is quick, active, powerful, and sharper than any double-edged sword and can reach into anywhere to effect healing.

Proverbs 18:20-21; Matthew8:8; Luke7:7- Speak only the word as you lay hands on them and they shall be healed in the Name of Jesus.

Teach the sick - the unconverted sick person, the newly born again sick person, the believer sick person the Living Word of God.

For the unconverted or newly born again, laying on of hands is the way for their healing. It is not the only way but is the major way to heal them and bring them over to the faith.

For the believer who belongs to the church and has elders who oversee them, calling on the elders, the prayer of faith and anointing with oil in the name of the Lord is the way to their healing! It is not the only way, but the major way ordained by the Lord to keep the believer healthy.

In all, it is The LORD who operates or acts in diverse ways to heal the sick, save them and raise them up. So FAITH and OBEDIENCE TO THE LIVING WORD is the basic requirement.

Unbelievers and Believers Must Have Faith in The Living Word

Unbelievers (John5:24) must have faith in The Living Word and believers (1John3:14) must obey The Living Word for both to be healed. (The write up is how to pass from death to life by all- unbelievers and Believers).

Faith is hearing and obeying God's Word
To Hear The Living Word and Believe it (have faith in it) or obey it is what faith is all about.
Romans 10:17- Faith cometh by hearing, and hearing by the Word of God.

Faith is believing and acting on God's Word
To hear and believe or act on The Living Word is what exercising faith is all about.
Healing is never in view unless the unconverted or newly born again believes The Living Word and the believer obeys it. It is man's FAITH AND OBEDIENCE TO THE LIVING WORD that commits the integrity and faithfulness of the Lord to make good His word by healing all of their sicknesses and diseases. Whether you are unconverted, newly converted or a believer,
Believe and obey The Living Word and nothing will stop your healing. Know what He expects you to do and do it and nothing, and no one will deny you your healing or blessing that you desire.

CHAPTER 5

DEMONSTRATING YOUR FAITH

How You Show and Demonstrate Your Faith

Have faith, testify or confess always what you believe to be the truth

Hebrew 10:19-23

19 ¶ Therefore, brethren, having boldness to enter the Holiest by the blood of Jesus,

20 by a new and living way which He consecrated for us, through the veil, that is, His flesh,

21 and having a High Priest over the house of God,

22 let us draw near with a true heart in full assurance of faith, having our hearts sprinkled from an evil conscience and our bodies washed with pure water.

23 Let us hold fast the confession of our hope without wavering, for He who promised is faithful.

Ever be joyful and thankful
1Thessalolians 5:16-18
16 ¶ Rejoice always,
 17 pray without ceasing,
 18 in everything give thanks; for this is the will of God in Christ Jesus for you.

Ever be praiseful and offer sacrifices
Hebrews 13:15-16
15 Therefore by Him let us continually offer the sacrifice of praise to God, that is, the fruit of our lips, giving thanks to His name.
 16 But do not forget to do good and to share, for with such sacrifices God is well pleased.

Ever share testimonies
Revelations 12:11 "And they overcame him by the blood of the Lamb and by the word of their testimony, and they did not love their lives to the death."
In spite of how you feel, give voice to your faith in thankfulness, praises and testimonies.

Disregard the symptoms, circumstances; feelings, outlooks, etc and focus all your attention on The Living Word and God who cannot lie. Focus all your attention on the living Word of God that cannot be altered or changed.

See your healing no matter what symptoms may be there because God says so.
Have hands been laid on you? Then you must recover.

Have you been anointed with oil in the Lord's Name? Then you must be healed, saved and raised up.

God cannot lie neither can He break His covenant nor alter the Word He has spoken. You will be healed and delivered in Jesus Name.

Heaven and earth may pass away, but His Word which is forever settled in heaven will never pass away.

Disobedience Destroys Believers

Isaiah 1:18-20
18 "Come now, and let us reason together," Says the LORD, "Though your sins are like scarlet, They shall be as white as snow; Though they are red like crimson, They shall be as wool.
 19 If you are willing and obedient, You shall eat the good of the land;
 20 But if you refuse and rebel, You shall be devoured by the sword"; For the mouth of the LORD has spoken.

Job 36:10-12
10 He also opens their ear to instruction, And commands that they turn from iniquity.
 11 If they obey and serve Him, They shall spend their days in prosperity, And their years in pleasures.
 12 But if they do not obey, They shall perish by the sword, And they shall die without knowledge.

Psalm 82:5-7

5 They do not know, nor do they understand; They walk about in darkness; All the foundations of the earth are unstable.

6 ¶ I said, "You are gods, And all of you are children of the Most High.

7 But you shall die like men, And fall like one of the princes."

Psalm 100:1-5

1 ¶ <<A Psalm of Thanksgiving.>> Make a joyful shout to the LORD, all you lands!

2 Serve the LORD with gladness; Come before His presence with singing.

3 Know that the LORD, He is God; It is He who has made us, and not we ourselves; We are His people and the sheep of His pasture.

4 Enter into His gates with thanksgiving, And into His courts with praise. Be thankful to Him, and bless His name.

5 For the LORD is good; His mercy is everlasting, And His truth endures to all generations.

James 5:14-15

14 Is anyone among you sick? Let him call for the elders of the church, and let them pray over him, anointing him with oil in the name of the Lord.

15 And the prayer of faith will save the sick, and the Lord will raise him up. And if he has committed sins, he will be forgiven.

The above Scriptures are clear commandments the Lord have given to us His chosen ones.

Sick believers die when they refuse to call for the Elders of the church to pray over them and anoint them in the Name of the Lord but rather chose or prefer to call medical doctors. Such acts are defiant disobedience to the statute, command, ordinance, word, law or covenant of God for the New Testament believers. The consequences may result in death or destruction.

Unbelief Destroys Unbelievers

Sick unbelievers and the newly born again die when they refuse to believe or have faith in The Living Word and accept their healing when hands have been laid on them. To choose to do anything else after hands have been laid on you is a demonstration of unbelief and can result in the death and destruction of the unbeliever or the newly converted.

HIV/AIDS will be terminated in the believer's life when he calls the elders and they speak the word of faith over him, pray and anoint him with the anointing oil in the name of the Lord. And so will all other incurable sicknesses and diseases.
HIV/AIDS will be terminated in the unconverted life or that of the new convert when believers lay hands on them by faith in the Name of the Lord Jesus. And so will all other incurable ailments, bodily afflictions, illness, sicknesses or diseases.

There is no sickness or disease that will remain in the body or life of the believer when he obeys The Living Word of God and invites the Pastors or Leaders of the church to do what God has commanded for the healing, emancipation and recovery of the sick believer regardless of their sickness and its cause. That means the word of faith and anointing with oil in the Name of the Lord Jesus Christ by the Pastors over the sick believer is what the Lord requires to put to an end all forms of afflictions in the body of believers. But they all must show their faith in God by calling on the Pastors, Leaders, Ministers in the church.

Have faith in God, call on the elders, let them pray over you and anoint you in the name of the Lord and you shall be saved and the Lord will raise you up and even if you have committed sins, you will be forgiven. This is at no cost. It is free. You are not to pay the way for the elders who are to come. All you need do is to call for them or send for them. You need not pay any consultation fee. All God require is your implicit faith in obedience to Him and His word. Are you a believer and sick? Call and be healed. Please be free to call on us if you can't get help from those around you. We are here for you.

"Anyone among you" could be anybody - the Bishop, Pastors, Elders or Ministers or members. No matter your portfolio, if you are a believer and a member of the church of God, you belong to God.

Are you sick? Don't be ashamed about it. Never let pride step in and destroy you. Have you sinned and are afflicted by the enemy with sickness? Or you just took ill yet you don't know the cause of it.

Is your faith going through trials to see whether you trust in the Lord with all your heart (Proverb 3:5-6) or you trust in men (doctors) or are proud?

What God expects you to do is to humble yourself and submit to His Word by calling on the Elders of the church and let them pray the prayer of faith and anoint you with oil in the name of the Lord and you shall be healed and saved; and the Lord will raise you up and even if you have committed sins, you will be forgiven.

Acts 10:34-38
34 ¶ Then Peter opened his mouth and said: "In truth I perceive that God shows no partiality.
35 "But in every nation whoever fears Him and works righteousness is accepted by Him.
36 "The word which God sent to the children of Israel, preaching peace through Jesus Christ--He is Lord of all--
37 "that word you know, which was proclaimed throughout all Judea, and began from Galilee after the baptism which John preached:
38 "how God anointed Jesus of Nazareth with the Holy Spirit and with power, who went about doing good and healing all who were oppressed by the devil, for God was with Him.

God is no respecter of persons. Whoever hearkens to him and acts in obedience to His revealed word shall be saved, healed and raised up and established. There is no difference.

Romans 3:22 says "the righteousness of God, through faith in Jesus Christ,{is} to all and on all who believe. For there is no difference."

Romans 10:11-13
11 For the Scripture says, "Whoever believes on Him will not be put to shame."

12 ¶ For there is no distinction between Jew and Greek, for the same Lord over all is rich to all who call upon Him.
 13 For "whoever calls on the name of the LORD shall be saved."

Galatians 3:28 There is neither Jew nor Greek, there is neither slave nor free, there is neither male nor female; for you are all one in Christ Jesus.

Colossians 3:11 "where there is neither Greek nor Jew, circumcised nor uncircumcised, barbarian, Scythian, slave nor free, but Christ is all and in all."

The Just Lives by Faith
The just cannot live without by faith.
Habakkuk 2:4 "Behold the proud, His soul is not upright in him; But the just shall live by his faith."
Hebrew 10:38-39
38 Now the just shall live by faith; But if anyone draws back, My soul has no pleasure in him."
 39 But we are not of those who draw back to perdition, but of those who believe to the saving of the soul.

Obey the Living Word of God and Live
Call on the elders if you are a believer no matter your rank in the church. It is better you walk in obedience and live rather than walk in disobedience and die or be destroyed.
No sickness is anything before the Lord.
All He desires and demands is faith and obedience to His commands. It gets Him committed to acting on your behalf.

Are you not born again and sick or newly converted yet sick, God wants you healed. All you need is for hands to be laid on you and the Lord will carry out His operations or activities to enforce your recovery or healing, no matter what your sickness may be.

All you need do is to submit to His Word. When you seek medicine first and not The Lord who is The Healer, you end in death.

Believers - the Israel of God according to Galatians 6:16 die when they consult false gods.

Ahaziah was sick and instead of consulting God, looking up to and obeying Him for his healing sent to consult a false god - the god of Ekron called Baalzebub and He died of his sickness (see 2Kings 1:2-4, 6, 16-17).

What Ahaziah did is the same believers do when they consult the gods of the world. God sent to him His messenger to tell him he will die for consulting a false god and not the Living God of Israel. And he died.

2Chronicles 16:12-13 Asa also died because he sought men and not the Lord.

God says in 1Timothy 6:20, "Science is false" which means it is unreliable.

CHAPTER 6

WHY NO SICK BELIEVER MUST DIE

Why No Sick Believer Must Die

In one Paul's ministrations a young man named Eutychus who sat listening to the Word fell from a 3-storey building. In fact he was found dead. But Paul went and embraced him where he laid on the ground floor dead and he came back to life.

Acts 20:7-12

7 ¶ Now on the first day of the week, when the disciples came together to break bread, Paul, ready to depart the next day, spoke to them and continued his message until midnight.

8 There were many lamps in the upper room where they were gathered together.

9 And in a window sat a certain young man named Eutychus, who was sinking into a deep sleep. He was overcome by sleep; and as Paul continued speaking, he fell down from the third story and was taken up dead.

10 But Paul went down, fell on him, and embracing him said, "Do not trouble yourselves, for his life is in him."

11 Now when he had come up, had broken bread and eaten, and talked a long while, even till daybreak, he departed.

12 And they brought the young man in alive, and they were not a little comforted.

Eutychus was restored back to life and he lived. That shows God wants you to live and not die to declare His works. But believers die sick. Why? What is/are the reason(s) why God's own children are not healed but die sick?

1. King Ahaziah died because he did not seek God.

2Kings 1:2-4, 6, 16-17

2 Now Ahaziah fell through the lattice of his upper room in Samaria, and was injured; so he sent messengers and said to them, "Go, inquire of Baal-Zebub, the god of Ekron, whether I shall recover from this injury."

3 But the angel of the LORD said to Elijah the Tishbite, "Arise, go up to meet the messengers of the king of Samaria, and say to them, 'Is it because there is no God in Israel that you are going to inquire of Baal-Zebub, the god of Ekron?'

4 "Now therefore, thus says the LORD: 'You shall not come down from the bed to which you have gone up, but you shall surely die.'" So Elijah departed.

6 So they said to him, "A man came up to meet us, and said to us, 'Go, return to the king who sent you, and say to him, "Thus says the LORD: 'Is it because there is no God in Israel that you are sending to inquire of Baal-Zebub, the god of Ekron? Therefore you shall not come down from the bed to which you have gone up, but you shall surely die.'"'"

16 Then he said to him, "Thus says the LORD: 'Because you have sent messengers to inquire of Baal-Zebub, the god of Ekron, is it because there is no God in Israel to inquire of His word? Therefore you shall not come down from the bed to which you have gone up, but you shall surely die.'"

17 So Ahaziah died according to the word of the LORD which Elijah had spoken.

Ahaziah fell off his upstairs room and was seriously injured and instead of seeking the Lord, he sought the god of Ekron (god of medicine). And God sent him the word that he must surely die for not seeking him and he died. If Ahaziah had sought the God of Israel, he would not have died.

2. Elisha died sick with all his Anointing

2 Kings 13:14, 20
14 Elisha had become sick with the illness of which he would die.
20 ¶ Then Elisha died, and they buried him.

He had a double portion of Elijah's anointing yet died sick. God is no respecter of persons. If you fail to accept His provisions for you, He won't force you to do otherwise. You can live and die like Elisha (**Read my book**: **"Why Prophet Elisha Died Sick"**).

3. King Asa died because he didn't seek the Lord.

2Chronicles 16:12-13
12 And in the thirty-ninth year of his reign, Asa became diseased in his feet, and his malady was severe; yet in his disease he did not seek the LORD, but the physicians.
13 So Asa rested with his fathers; he died in the forty-first year of his reign.

Asa was diseased in his feet but instead of seeking the Lord, he sought help from the physicians or doctors. So he died!

Asa was Jehoshaphat's father but died because he sought the help of doctors when he was sick and diseased and not the Lord our healer.

From Ahaziah and Asa's cases, it is very clear that when God's people abandon Him and go in search of men, doctors, physicians for help in times of sickness, disease, or illness, they end up suffering or dying.

Anointing With Oil Rescued The Sick
James 5:14-15
14 Is anyone among you sick? Let him call for the elders of the church, and let them pray over him, anointing him with oil in the name of the Lord.
 15 And the prayer of faith will save the sick, and the Lord will raise him up. And if he has committed sins, he will be forgiven.

No matter the stage of sickness, even if the sick cannot move again but lies at the point of death, God says, call on the elders. Obey.

Mark 6:12-13
12 So they went out and preached that people should repent.
 13 And they cast out many demons, and anointed with oil many who were sick, and healed them.

The apostles anointed the sick with oil in the Name of the Lord and healed every one of them. The anointing with oil in the Name of the Lord plus the prayer of faith got the sick healed and saved. The Lord [by Himself] raised them up; and if they had committed sins, they were forgiven.

Proclaiming the Word Holds the Key to Healing

Psalm 107:20
20 He sent His word and healed them, And delivered them from their destructions.

Mark 16:15-18,

15 And He said to them, "Go into all the world and preach the gospel to every creature.

16 "He who believes and is baptized will be saved; but he who does not believe will be condemned.

17 "And these signs will follow those who believe: In My name they will cast out demons; they will speak with new tongues;

18 "they will take up serpents; and if they drink anything deadly, it will by no means hurt them; they will lay hands on the sick, and they will recover."

Acts 14:7-10

7 And they were preaching the gospel there.

8 ¶ And in Lystra a certain man without strength in his feet was sitting, a cripple from his mother's womb, who had never walked.

9 This man heard Paul speaking. Paul, observing him intently and seeing that he had faith to be healed,

10 said with a loud voice, "Stand up straight on your feet!" And he leaped and walked.

Paul the believer did it also in Acts 20:7-12. Paul preached and when death struck Paul humiliated it by faith and the dead came back to life.

Mark 16:19-20

19 ¶ So then, after the Lord had spoken to them, He was received up into heaven, and sat down at the right hand of God.

20 And they went out and preached everywhere, the Lord working with them and confirming the word through the accompanying signs. Amen.

Believers who ignore this command of the Lord and go in search of medicine and doctors as both Ahaziah and Asa did respectively will end up in much suffering. God's word is very clear about it.

But note: You get the Lord committed to validating His Word when you believe and obey His Word. Why seek men and destroy yourself? Ahaziah and Asa sought men and so died of their diseases and sicknesses. May you not end as they ended.

Examples of Those Who Sought The Lord
And What Happened To Them

1. King Benhaded Recovered because he sought the Lord.
2Kings 8:7-10, 14*(RSV)*
7 Now Elisha came to Damascus. Benhadad the king of Syria was sick, and when it was told him, "the man of God has come here,"
8 The king said to Hazael, "Take a present with you and go to meet the man of God, and inquire of the Lord through him, saying, shall I recover from this sickness?"
9 So Hazael went to meet him, and took a present with him, all kinds of goods of Damascus, forty Camel loads. When he came and stood before him, he said, "Your son Benhaded king of Syria has sent me to you, saying, 'shall I recover from this sickness?'
10 And Elisha said to him, "Go say to him, You shall certainly recover",
14 Then he departed from Elisha, and came to his master, who said to him, "What did Elisha say to you?" And he answered, "He told me that you would certainly recover."

King Benhaded sought the Lord and the word of the Lord went forth to him, "You shall certainly recover."

Proverb 4:22 shows that The Living Word is life to those who finds it and health (medicine) to all their flesh.

Isaiah 45:22-23

22 "Look to Me, and be saved, All you ends of the earth! For I am God, and there is no other.

23 I have sworn by Myself; The word has gone out of My mouth in righteousness, And shall not return, That to Me every knee shall bow, Every tongue shall take an oath.

Isaiah 55:8-12

8 "For My thoughts are not your thoughts, Nor are your ways My ways," says the LORD.

9 "For as the heavens are higher than the earth, So are My ways higher than your ways, And My thoughts than your thoughts.

10 "For as the rain comes down, and the snow from heaven, And do not return there, But water the earth, And make it bring forth and bud, That it may give seed to the sower And bread to the eater,

11 So shall My word be that goes forth from My mouth; It shall not return to Me void, But it shall accomplish what I please, And it shall prosper in the thing for which I sent it.

12 "For you shall go out with joy, And be led out with peace...

The Living Word He sent cannot fail to accomplish the very purpose God sent it to accomplish. Therefore, The Living Word from the Lord to king Benhaded brought healing to him.

Psalm 107:20 "He sent His word and healed them and delivered them from their destructions."

The Word of the LORD to Benhaded was that He will recover. And he did, but the next day, he died, not by the sickness but at the hands of his servant - Hazael who assassinated him and took over the throne. God wants to heal all. See also John 4:49-53; Matthew 8:5, 6, 13; Mark 7:24-30; Luke7:1-10.

2. King Hezekiah lived because he sought the Lord.

2 Kings 20:1-6 *(RSV)*
1 In those days Hezekiah became sick and was at the point of death.
And Isaiah the prophet the son of Amoz came to him, "Thus says the Lord, 'set your house in order; for you shall die, you shall not recover!"
2 Then Hezekiah turned his face to the wall and prayed to the Lord, saying,
3 "Remember now, O Lord, I beseech thee, how I have walked before thee in faithfulness and with a whole heart, and have done what is good in thy sight." And Hezekiah wept bitterly.
4 And before Isaiah had gone out of the middle court, the word of the Lord came to him:
5 Turn back, and say to Hezekiah the prince of my people, Thus says the Lord, the God of David your father: I have heard your prayer, I have seen your tears; behold, I will heal you; on the 3rd day you shall go up to the house of the Lord.
6 And I will add fifteen (15) years to your life.

From the point of death, Hezekiah sought the Lord and not only was he healed but 15 more years were added to him. Hezekiah's health and recovery was perfected and within three (3) days at the house of the Lord. *See Isaiah 38:1-10*

Two kings died for not seeking God but men
- King Ahaziah of Israel died for not seeking the Lord.
- King Assa of Judah died for not seeking the Lord.

Two kings Recovered for seeking God

• King Benhaded of Syria lived because he sought the Lord God.
• King Hezekiah of Judah lived because he sought the Lord

Four of them were kings (Israel/Samaria, Judah, Syria, Judah).

Revelation 5:9-10 shows We are kings and priests.
Two (2) kings died for failing to seek the Lord for their healing when they were sick.
Two (2) kings recovered for seeking the Lord for their healing when they were sick.
Believers may end like the 2 kings that died when they fail to seek the Lord for their healing. But we will live when we seek the Lord for healing.

New Testament Examples
1. The Centurions servant who was sick and at the point of death, got healed and delivered from destruction because they sought the Lord on his behalf.

Matthew 8:5-8, 13

5 ¶ Now when Jesus had entered Capernaum, a centurion came to Him, pleading with Him,

6 saying, "Lord, my servant is lying at home paralyzed, dreadfully tormented."

7 And Jesus said to him, "I will come and heal him."

8 The centurion answered and said, "Lord, I am not worthy that You should come under my roof. But only speak a word, and my servant will be healed.

13 Then Jesus said to the centurion, "Go your way; and as you have believed, so let it be done for you." And his servant was healed that same hour. *(See Luke 7:1-10; Psalm 107:20)*

2. The official's son who was ill got healed and delivered from his destruction because they sought the Lord for his healing.

John 4:46-53

46 So Jesus came again to Cana of Galilee where He had made the water wine. And there was a certain nobleman whose son was sick at Capernaum.

47 When he heard that Jesus had come out of Judea into Galilee, he went to Him and implored Him to come down and heal his son, for he was at the point of death.

48 Then Jesus said to him, "Unless you people see signs and wonders, you will by no means believe."

49 The nobleman said to Him, "Sir, come down before my child dies!"

50 Jesus said to him, "Go your way; your son lives." So the man believed the word that Jesus spoke to him, and he went his way.

51 And as he was now going down, his servants met him and told him, saying, "Your son lives!"

52 Then he inquired of them the hour when he got better. And they said to him, "Yesterday at the seventh hour the fever left him."

53 So the father knew that it was at the same hour in which Jesus said to him, "Your son lives." And he himself believed, and his whole household.

You don't need to suffer the fate of the ignorant. They die like men and fall like one of the princes (see Psalm 82:5-7).

Live and reign!

CHAPTER 7

THE KEY TO LIFE AND HEALTH

"Search from the book of the LORD, and read: Not one of these shall fail... For My mouth has commanded it, and His Spirit has gathered them. *Isaiah 34:16*

Proverb 4:20-22

20 ¶ My son, give attention to my words; Incline your ear to my sayings.

21 Do not let them depart from your eyes; Keep them in the midst of your heart;

22 For they are life to those who find them, And health to all their flesh.

Beware: Don't be Lazy

"By MUCH slothfulness the building decayeth; and through idleness of the hands the House droppeth through." *Ecclesiastes 10:18*

Slothfulness is Laziness. It is Idleness. The Building or The House or The Temple (which temple 'You' are if you are born again - 1Corinthians 3:16), or the Body of Christ decays as a result of sickness because of laziness.

As God's building, everything you need to be healthy and preserved body, soul and spirit is in The Living Word.

The Living Word is health or medicine for all your flesh. The Living Word is Life to them who find it. The NIV says, "they The Living Word, are life to those who find them and Health to a man's whole body."

Man is a tripartite being. Man is a Spirit, has a Soul and lives in a body.

The Living Word keeps the Spirit, Soul and body of man alive and healthy when he finds it.

The Living Word when received into a man's spirit creates a new man and keeps the Spirit alive.

The Living Word keeps the soul alive and healthy when man thinks on The Living Word.

The Living Word keeps the body alive and healthy when man Acts on The Living Word.

To Receive, Think on or Act on The Living Word is WORK.
Reading the Scripture is Work (1Timothy 4:13, 15).
Studying The Living Word is Work (2Timothy 2:15).
Searching the Scripture is work (John5:39). Meditating on the Word is work (Joshua 1:8).

Acting on The Living Word is serious work. To be lazy in Reading, Studying, Searching or Acting on The Living Word is the easiest way to position you for destruction.

Ecclesiastes 10:18, "By much slothfulness (laziness) the Building (God's house or temple, which temple you are) decayeth; and through idleness of hands (Hands represents Doing or Acting on The Living Word), the house (Temple/You) droppeth through."

To be healed and live healthy, The Living Word must be completely Read, Studied, Meditated, Received and Acted on. Then life and health will be the product (Proverb 4:20-22; John 6:63)

Hosea 4:6 says God's people are destroyed for lack of knowledge.
Isaiah 5:13 says God's people walk into sickness, disease, captivity because they have no knowledge.
Psalm 82:7 Gods die like men and fall like Satan (one of the princes-see Luke 10:18) because they know not, neither do they understand.

To learn, have knowledge and understand is not for lazy men.

The ants keep moving and are kept healthy and preserved always.

Learn from the ants to keep working and labouring in the Word of God and you'll be preserved in life and health and live healthy. See Proverb 6:4-11, Proverb 24:30-3.

The easiest way to end in captivity, sickness, disease, poverty is to ignore The Living Word or to fail to labour in the word always. Be an addicted and committed reader and student of the Word and life from The Living Word will be your portion.

Proverb 4:20-22

20 ¶ My son, give attention to my words; Incline your ear to my sayings.

21 Do not let them depart from your eyes; Keep them in the midst of your heart;

22 For they are life to those who find them, And health to all their flesh.

2Timothy 2:15 15 Be diligent to present yourself approved to God, a worker who does not need to be ashamed, rightly dividing the word of truth.

1Timothy 4:13, 15

13 Till I come, give attention to reading, to exhortation, to doctrine.

15 Meditate on these things; give yourself entirely to them, that your progress may be evident to all.

Joshua 1:8 "This Book of the Law shall not depart from your mouth, but you shall meditate in it day and night, that you may observe to do according to all that is written in it. For then you will make your way prosperous, and then you will have good success.

Ecclesiastes 9:10 "Whatever your hand finds to do, do it with your might; for there is no work or device or knowledge or wisdom in the grave where you are going."

Proverb 10:14 ¶ Wise people store up knowledge, But the mouth of the foolish is near destruction.

Daniel Read and Lived

Daniel 9:2 shows that Daniel read and lived so long that he served under 3 Kings of Babylon and continued long after they were all gone (Daniel 1;21; 2Chronicles 36:22; Daniel 6:28; 10:1).
He lived until the predictions of God through the Prophets that lived long before Daniel's time were fulfilled. He didn't see death because he knew what was to happen from the book.

Hezekiah Read and Lived

Hezekiah read and knew how long he was to live and when God said he was to die, he asked God to let him live up to the exact number of years God has allotted to him. God bound by His Word caused sickness to be cleared off his life and the remainder of his years (15 years) was added. See Isaiah 38:10, 2-9.

Paul Read and Lived

Paul read and heard God's Word very clearly and lived to fulfill his days until he finished his work and was ready to go. (Deuteronomy 30:15, 19-20; 2Timothy 4:13; Philippians 1:21-26; Proverbs 18:21; Psalm 118:17).

You Can Read and Live!
Isaiah 34:16 "Search from the book of the LORD, and read: Not one of these shall fail... For My mouth has commanded it, and His Spirit has gathered them."

In Exodus 23:26 The Lord says, "the number of thy days I will fulfill."

Understand your legal rights and privileges as provided in the Living Word of God and ask God for them. And you'll have them.

You can be free of sickness, disease, poverty, plagues and all evil. All you need is to know what is available in The Living Word and ask God for it and it will be delivered. What you can search out from the book of promise is yours. You must not allow yourself or any other believer to die in his or her sickness.

You have been healed!

1 Peter 2:24, "who Himself bore our sins in His own body on the tree, that we, having died to sins, might live for righteousness--by whose stripes you were healed."
"By whose stripes you were healed." You have been healed! The Lord says so.

See what is yours and take it. That's why the Book of Life is packaged and given to us.

Don't be lazy. Don't be slothful. Don't be idle. Don't destroy the building (you) or the house of God by being lazy or idle.

Healing/Health are Available: Go For It!

Healing is available. Better still, health is available. You must learn what you have to learn so that you can have what is yours. This is wisdom.

No more decay for you. You shall no longer drop through because of idleness. Nothing about your life will be wasted nor trampled underfoot by the wicked.

Learn. Acquire Knowledge and Skill

Read, 1Timothy4:13, 15; Isaiah 34:16.

Study, 2 Timothy 2:15.

Search, John5:39; Isaiah 34:16.

Meditate, Psalm 1:2-3; Philippians 4:8.

Speak, Proverb 4:20-22, Proverb18:21.

Be diligent, Joshua 1:8; Proverbs 22:29.

Act or do what you've discovered from The Living Word. Every chain of evil tying you down must drop off your life in Jesus Name.

Daniel outlived three (3) kings of Babylon because of His Commitment to READING.

Hezekiah and Paul did too.

John 1:1-3

1 ¶ In the beginning was the Word, and the Word was with God, and the Word was God.

2 He was in the beginning with God.

3 All things were made through Him, and without Him nothing was made that was made.

John 6:63 "It is the Spirit who gives life; the flesh profits nothing. The words that I speak to you are spirit, and they are life."

Romans 12:1-2
1 ¶ I beseech you therefore, brethren, by the mercies of God, that you present your bodies a living sacrifice, holy, acceptable to God, which is your reasonable service.
2 And do not be conformed to this world, but be transformed by the renewing of your mind, that you may prove what is that good and acceptable and perfect will of God.

Ephesians 4:23-24
23 and be renewed in the spirit of your mind,
24 and that you put on the new man which was created according to God, in true righteousness and holiness.

Deuteronomy 30:14-20
14 "But the word is very near you, in your mouth and in your heart, that you may do it.
15 ¶ "See, I have set before you today life and good, death and evil,
16 "in that I command you today to love the LORD your God, to walk in His ways, and to keep His commandments, His statutes, and His judgments, that you may live and multiply; and the LORD your God will bless you in the land which you go to possess.

17 "But if your heart turns away so that you do not hear, and are drawn away, and worship other gods and serve them,

18 "I announce to you today that you shall surely perish; you shall not prolong your days in the land which you cross over the Jordan to go in and possess.

19 "I call heaven and earth as witnesses today against you, that I have set before you life and death, blessing and cursing; therefore choose life, that both you and your descendants may live;

20 "that you may love the LORD your God, that you may obey His voice, and that you may cling to Him, for He is your life and the length of your days; and that you may dwell in the land which the LORD swore to your fathers, to Abraham, Isaac, and Jacob, to give them."

When Your Mind is filled with life from The Living Word, your body will live because as He thinks, so he is (Proverbs 23:7). And as he speaks and does, so he becomes and possesses (Proverbs 18:21; Joshua 1:8; Psalm 1:3).
Read. Think. Speak as God does always!
Think on the Word. Speak the Word. And Live the Word. The Word is God. God is The Word. When you get the revelation of the Word and Live by it, you will live exactly as God Lives! Peace always and by all means is yours! It's a new day for you.

I am expecting your testimonies.

Please write and share your testimonies with us.

If You are not certain that You are Born Again as you are certain about your name, or You were once saved but went astray again, living and doing as you pleased, Then say aloud this Prayer:

PRAYER FOR SALVATION AND RESTORATION!

Dear Heavenly Father, I return to you by Faith. I am sorry for my sins. I believe in my heart Jesus is The Christ and that He died for my sins and rose from the dead on the third day, according to Scripture, for my justification. I confess that Jesus Christ is LORD and I accept Him now as my Saviour. I believe my sins are wiped away.
I call upon The Name of The LORD for my total Healing, Liberty and Restoration.
I ask for the Gift of Your Holy Spirit, Power and Grace to follow and serve You from this day forward. And I Thank You Abba Father for doing far beyond all I have asked and can ever imagine in Jesus Name. Amen!
I NOW DECLARE THAT I AM A CHILD OF GOD FOREVER!

You can also Enlist now and become a Partner and or Member of our Totally Empowered Ambassadors on Mission (TEAM) and see what Our Risen Lord and King Jesus Christ will transform your life into and do in, for and through you from this day as believe and obey His Word!

For further enquiries

Send an E-mail or visit our website:

Amb Promise Ogbonna

Christ's Ambassadors Living Mission Int'l - *Jesus Mission Headquarters*

WhatsApp or Text: **+2348060635805, +2348053995257, +2348027829586**

E-mail: ambpromiseo@gmail.com

CHRIST'S AMBASSADORS LIVING MISSION INT'L - *JESUS MISSION HEADQUARTERS*

WELCOMES YOU TO THESE SPECIALIZED SERVICES

Weekdays: 12:00-1:00pm. Hour of EmPowerment for All
Saturdays: 8:00-9:00am. Hour of Healing & Freedom for All
Sundays: 8:00-9:00am. Hour of Liberty & Restoration for All
Sundays: 9:00-10:00am. Hour of Kingdom Wealth Transfer to All
Last Friday Night Monthly: 10:00pm. Night of Restorations for All
Ambassadors Bible Institute: Trains and Releases Christ's Ambassadors on His Mission everywhere! Enroll today!

Venue: 24 Independence Street, Behind O'MARK Schools by O'MARK Bus Stop, LASU Road, Igando Lagos.

<u>**ABOUT THE AUTHOR**</u>

The Risen Lord Jesus Christ appointed and commissioned Amb Promise Ogbonna as His Official Ambassador and Living Witness and sent him with His Staff of Office to Prove to all worldwide that He is ALIVE TODAY! He is sent to Proclaim and Publish The Everlasting Gospel to every creature everywhere; To Stop anything after man's destruction; To Bring Healing, Liberty and Restoration to all; To Raise, Build and Plant all as Christ's Ambassadors on His Mission everywhere and Restore all things at all cost and by all means!

He is the President of Christ's Ambassadors Living Mission International Inc., an all-encompassing network of ministries and Lead Pastor of CHRIST'S AMBASSADORS - JESUS MISSION HEADQUARTERS, a non-denominational Assembly and Fellowship of Ambassadors and Citizens of Heaven on Christ's Mission worldwide.

He is married to Favour Promise, a trained Lawyer and they are blessed with four wonderful children.

OUR HEALING PRODUCTS AND SERVICES
1. All-Purpose Divine Healing Medicine
2. Healing Messages - CD, MP3 & DVD

3. Healing Books
4. Healing Leaves Magazine
5. Healing Anointing Oil
6. Healing Mantles & Clothes
7. Healing Materials
8. Healing Elixir for incurable diseases
9. Healing Songs
10. Healing Homes
11. Healing Seminars
12. Healing School
13. Healing Teams
14. Healing Outreaches & Explosions
15. World Healing Conferences
16. Health Centre
17. Healing Balm

We are on a Mission to free the World from all sicknesses and diseases and Restore ALL to God's Original Condition, Plan, Place and Purpose!

Call us now for our Healing Products and Services! We can't wait to SERVE YOU!

OTHER BOOKS BY AMB PROMISE OGBONNA
1. The Nothingness of Satan
2. You Can Make a Fresh Start
3. Restoring The Forgotten Dignity of Woman
4. Christ's Ambassadors: Raising Rulers in God's Own Very Class
5. Christ's Ambassadors: Building Rulers in God's Own Very Class
6. Christ's Ambassadors: Re-Emergence of Rulers in God's Own Very Class
**Christ's Ambassadors: Re-Emergence of Rulers in God's Own Very Class Handbook
7. Manifesting As Signs and Wonders.

8. 40 Pitfalls to Avoid.
9. Wisdom Seeds to Greatness In Life
10. Why Prophet Elisha Died Sick and how to Avoid it
11. You Can Choose When to Die
12. You Shall Live and Not Die
13. Why Christians Die Sick…
14. 7 Keys to Undeniable Healing
15. 8 Decisive Hours That Will Take You To The Topmost